UNDERSTANDING

THREAD LIFTS THERAPY

FOR BEGINNERS

Discover Advanced Techniques, Client Care Strategies, And Expert Insights For Achieving Safe And Effective Non-Surgical Facelifts

DR. ALICIA SONYA

CONTENTS

DISCLAIMER

The information provided in this book is for educational and informational purposes only and is not intended as medical advice, diagnosis, or treatment. Always consult with a qualified healthcare professional before beginning any therapy, practice, or lifestyle change.

The author and publisher of this book make no representations or warranties regarding the accuracy, applicability, or completeness of the content presented. While every effort has been made to ensure the information provided is accurate and up-to-date, the field of health and wellness is constantly evolving, and the reader is advised to use discretion and seek professional guidance as needed.

This book contains references to individuals, products, websites, organizations, or other entities solely for informational purposes. The author and publisher do not endorse, sponsor, or affiliate with any of these references, nor do they receive any benefit from their inclusion. The mention of any names, trademarks, or products does not imply any association or endorsement.

The use of this book is solely at the reader's discretion. Neither the author nor the publisher shall be held liable for any damages, loss, or injury resulting from the use or misuse of the information contained herein.

ABOUT THIS BOOK

Understanding Thread Lifts Therapy For Beginners" offers an essential resource for both seasoned practitioners and newcomers to the field of non-surgical facelifts, combining detailed knowledge of thread lift techniques with best practices for client care. Thread lifts, an increasingly popular alternative to traditional facelifts, provide a minimally invasive way to achieve facial rejuvenation with less recovery time, fewer risks, and customizable results.

This book begins by exploring the science behind thread lifts, breaking down the unique types of threads—PDO, PLLA, and PCL—each suited for specific effects and longevity.

Practitioners will also gain a deep understanding of facial anatomy, with emphasis on skin layers that interact with threads for optimal lift and sculpting. With attention to client goals and realistic outcomes, the book sets a strong foundation for delivering results that meet or exceed client expectations.

Preparation is critical in any aesthetic procedure, and this book provides comprehensive guidelines for consulting with clients, from assessing candidacy to educating them on the importance of sterilization and hygiene. Step-by-step pre-treatment care helps minimize risks, while an organized checklist of materials and equipment ensures readiness for each procedure.

For practitioners, this section reinforces the importance of a meticulous and hygienic environment, which supports both client safety and optimal results.

In its technique-focused sections, this book details the nuanced steps involved in thread insertion, offering insights into the differences between lifting and smooth threads.

Readers will find guidance on selecting the most effective methods for different facial areas, combining treatments for enhanced outcomes, and ensuring safe, complication-free procedures.

Anatomical considerations are woven throughout, with a dedicated exploration of the muscles, nerves, and vessels most relevant to threading. This anatomical knowledge equips practitioners to assess a client's facial structure accurately and create highly personalized results while helping to minimize risks associated with thread placement.

Post-procedure care is a critical aspect of long-term success in thread lift therapy, and this guide provides thorough protocols for immediate and extended care, covering everything from managing swelling to advising clients on activity restrictions.

Practitioners will appreciate the guidance on handling side effects, sustaining results, and setting up a reliable follow-up schedule to support client satisfaction. Clear guidelines for identifying and managing common complications, such as asymmetry, infection, or thread migration, empower practitioners to handle any concerns with confidence, ensuring safe and professional outcomes for each client.

For practitioners looking to refine their skills, this book introduces advanced techniques that can elevate results, such as combining different types of threads, using layering and angling for specific effects, and enhancing thread lifts with complementary treatments like fillers.

This advanced insight is supported by case studies that illustrate various applications, equipping readers with practical examples of high-level approaches. The section on client communication underscores the importance of trust and transparency in aesthetics, offering strategies for setting clear expectations, addressing questions, and ensuring satisfaction.

This book concludes with industry insights and best practices, covering critical trends in non-surgical facelifting and providing tips on certification, ethical practices, and business growth in aesthetics. Practitioners are encouraged to pursue continuous learning, maintain a strong foundation of current knowledge, and adapt to the latest developments in thread lift therapy.

As a comprehensive guide, this book equips aesthetic professionals to excel in thread lifts, from technique mastery to fostering meaningful client relationships and establishing a successful, trustworthy practice.

CHAPTER ONE

Understanding Thread Lifts

Thread lifts are a minimally invasive cosmetic procedure designed to lift and tighten sagging facial skin without surgery. Using temporary sutures, a specialist lifts portions of the skin to create a more youthful appearance. Thread lifts stimulate collagen production as the body responds to the threads, creating a natural tightening and firmness over time. This treatment is popular among those seeking subtle enhancements without the downtime and recovery associated with traditional facelifts.

In the procedure, a professional inserts dissolvable threads through small incisions in the targeted area.

These threads act as anchors that lift the skin while promoting healing and rejuvenation. Over time, the threads dissolve, but their effects last as collagen builds up around them. Areas commonly treated include the neck, jawline, cheeks, and eyebrows, though other areas can also benefit from this treatment.

Results from thread lifts vary based on individual skin characteristics, thread type, and technique, generally lasting 12 to 18 months. This therapy offers a gradual, natural improvement, appealing to individuals who prefer subtle, progressive results. Maintenance sessions can extend the effects, with practitioners recommending treatments every year or two to maintain optimal outcomes.

Overview Of Non-Surgical Facelifts And Thread Lift Therapy

Non-surgical facelifts focus on restoring youthful facial contours without invasive surgery. Thread lift therapy specifically uses specialized sutures to lift, reposition, and support areas of the face that have lost elasticity and firmness. Unlike surgical facelifts, thread lifts have minimal downtime, making them ideal for those who cannot commit to a long recovery period.

The treatment typically takes less than an hour, and local anesthesia is used to minimize discomfort. Threads are inserted through a fine needle or cannula, securing tissue in a lifted position. As the threads dissolve over several months, they encourage collagen growth, which helps to maintain the lift even after the threads have fully dissolved.

Thread lifts are not meant to replace a surgical facelift but provide a temporary, less intensive solution for early signs of aging. Individuals with moderate skin laxity and realistic expectations about subtle changes tend to see the best results. For deeper folds or significant sagging, a surgical facelift might be a more effective option.

Types Of Threads (PDO, PLLA, PCL) And Their Uses

There are three main types of threads used in thread lift procedures: PDO (polydioxanone), PLLA (poly-L-lactic acid), and PCL (polycaprolactone). PDO threads are among the most widely used for their durability and ability to stimulate collagen production. These threads dissolve within about six months, leaving a collagen scaffold that supports the skin for 12 to 18 months post-treatment.

PLLA threads are slightly more durable and offer longer-lasting results compared to PDO threads, taking around 12 months to dissolve. They are particularly effective in building collagen and are often used in deeper layers for more significant lifting. PCL threads are the most durable, dissolving over 24 months or more, providing sustained collagen support and enhanced lifting for extended results.

Choosing the right type of thread depends on the desired outcome, the area being treated, and the patient's unique skin type. Experienced practitioners assess each client's needs to determine the best option, often combining different types for optimal results. The customization allows for a tailored approach to lifting and contouring various parts of the face.

Key Benefits Of Thread Lifts Compared To Surgical Facelifts

Thread lifts offer a range of benefits over traditional facelifts, particularly for those looking for a less invasive option with minimal downtime.

The procedure itself is quick, typically under an hour, and can be performed in a clinic setting under local anesthesia, allowing clients to resume daily activities shortly after. The reduced recovery time appeals to those with busy lifestyles or commitments that prevent extended time away.

In addition to the lifting effect, thread lifts stimulate collagen production, providing gradual improvements in skin tone and texture. Unlike surgical facelifts, thread lifts do not leave noticeable scars as only small puncture points are made, which heal quickly. The natural lift provided by threads also allows for more subtle changes, creating a refreshed appearance without drastic alterations.

Thread lifts are significantly less expensive than surgical facelifts, making them accessible to a wider audience. Although the effects are not permanent, maintenance sessions can help extend results, making this a flexible option for clients seeking a more youthful look without the commitment and cost of surgery.

Basic Anatomy Of Facial Skin Layers Relevant To Thread Lifts

Thread lifts target specific facial layers to achieve a lifted and rejuvenated look. The skin consists of several layers: the epidermis (outermost), dermis (middle), and subcutaneous tissue (deepest). The dermis is where collagen and elastin fibers are found, which are essential for skin firmness and elasticity. During a thread lift, threads are positioned primarily in the subcutaneous layer to create the lifting effect while stimulating collagen production.

Practitioners insert threads at an angle and depth that optimally engages the skin's supportive structures, ensuring that the threads anchor properly and provide lift without affecting the surrounding tissue. Targeting the subcutaneous layer is essential because this layer is rich in collagen-producing cells, enabling the stimulation of new collagen as the threads dissolve.

Understanding these layers is crucial for practitioners, as incorrect thread placement can result in suboptimal outcomes or even complications.

Proper depth and alignment ensure the threads work harmoniously with the skin's natural structure, creating a smooth, lifted appearance without affecting muscle movements or expressions.

Understanding Client Expectations And Setting Realistic Goals

Achieving client satisfaction in thread lift therapy starts with setting realistic expectations. Before the procedure, practitioners hold consultations to discuss potential results, helping clients understand that thread lifts offer subtle, natural-looking enhancement rather than a dramatic facelift effect. Those seeking significant changes should consider that thread lifts provide moderate lifting and are best suited for early signs of aging.

During the consultation, clients review before-and-after photos to gain an understanding of achievable outcomes. This is the ideal time for practitioners to address individual skin concerns, such as sagging or fine lines, and to explain how these may be improved with thread lifts. Clear communication helps to avoid unrealistic expectations and ensures clients are fully informed.

Post-procedure, clients are advised to avoid heavy facial movements and specific skincare routines for a few days to optimize results. By setting clear, manageable expectations, practitioners foster a positive experience, as clients are more likely to be satisfied with their subtle, refreshed appearance when they understand the nature of thread lift therapy.

CHAPTER TWO

Preparing For A Thread Lift Procedure

Key Assessment And Consultation Steps

Before beginning a thread lift procedure, a comprehensive consultation is essential. During this meeting, the practitioner assesses the client's skin type, elasticity, and specific areas of concern, such as sagging cheeks, jowls, or neck. This discussion helps in tailoring the treatment to meet individual expectations. Moreover, the practitioner explains the benefits, limitations, and potential outcomes of a thread lift to set realistic expectations.

After discussing the client's goals, the practitioner examines the facial structure to identify the best areas for thread placement. Digital imaging or photographs may be taken to document the current state for before-and-after comparisons.

Additionally, it's important to note skin thickness, as this can influence the type of thread and technique used.

An individualized treatment plan is created, and the practitioner may recommend combining the thread lift with other non-surgical procedures, such as dermal fillers, to enhance the outcome.

By the end of the consultation, the client should clearly understand the procedure steps, anticipated results, and aftercare requirements.

Identifying Contraindications And Ideal Candidates

Thread lifts are suitable for individuals experiencing mild to moderate sagging who want a subtle lift without invasive surgery. Ideal candidates generally have good skin quality and are between 30 and 60 years old. However, people with severe sagging or extremely thin skin may not achieve optimal results and may need to consider alternative procedures.

Contraindications for thread lifts include active skin infections, uncontrolled diabetes, autoimmune disorders, or any coagulation or bleeding issues. Patients with known allergies to the materials used in the threads, such as polydioxanone (PDO) or polylactic acid (PLA), should avoid this procedure.

Additionally, people on blood thinners or those with a history of keloid scarring may need alternative options.

A thorough medical history review ensures that any health conditions, allergies, or current medications that could impact the procedure are identified. The practitioner can then decide if a thread lift is suitable or recommend other treatments to align with the client's health and aesthetic needs.

Client Preparation: Pre-Treatment Care Guidelines

Clients must follow specific pre-treatment guidelines to maximize the procedure's effectiveness and minimize side effects. Practitioners usually advise clients to avoid blood-thinning medications, alcohol, and certain supplements like Vitamin E, fish oil, or aspirin for about a week before the procedure, as these can increase the risk of bruising.

Skincare adjustments, such as avoiding retinoids and exfoliants, are also recommended in the days leading up to the appointment to reduce skin sensitivity. Clients should also avoid tanning, excessive sun exposure, or harsh skin treatments, as these can affect skin quality and increase irritation post-treatment.

On the day of the procedure, clients are advised to arrive with a clean face, free from makeup, lotions, or skincare products. Comfortable clothing, especially something that does not need to be pulled over the head, is suggested, as this minimizes friction around the treated areas after the procedure.

Importance Of Sterilization And Hygiene In The Procedure

Hygiene is paramount in thread lifting to prevent infection, as the procedure involves inserting threads beneath the skin. Practitioners must maintain a sterile environment, which includes sterilizing the treatment area, hands, and equipment. The client's skin is cleaned thoroughly with antiseptics before any threads are inserted, and a topical or local anesthetic is often applied to reduce discomfort.

The practitioner must wear gloves and use sterile tools throughout the procedure, and the threads themselves should be prepackaged and sterile. Any disposable items, such as syringes or gauze, are discarded immediately after use to prevent contamination.

After placing the threads, practitioners often apply an antibiotic ointment to reduce the risk of infection. Clients are advised not to touch or rub the treated area immediately following the procedure to maintain the sterile environment and reduce irritation.

Equipment And Materials Checklist For Thread Lifts

Practitioners performing thread lifts need specific equipment and materials to ensure safety and precision. Key items include pre-sterilized lifting threads, syringes, needles, gauze, antiseptic solutions, and local anesthetics. The threads used are typically either PDO, PLA, or PCL, which are absorbable and help stimulate collagen production over time. A clean, comfortable examination chair is necessary for client positioning, while good lighting aids in precise thread placement. Practitioners also need sterilized forceps, retractors, and marking pens to outline the targeted areas and secure the threads properly.

Finally, the practitioner should have a stock of post-treatment materials, such as antibiotic ointments and ice packs, for immediate aftercare. It's critical to check that all materials are present and in working order before starting the procedure to avoid interruptions and maintain a smooth, sterile process.

CHAPTER THREE

Thread Lift Techniques And Methods

Thread lifts employ different techniques and materials, depending on the desired outcome and the area being treated. The procedure generally uses two main types of threads: lifting threads, which are designed with barbs or cones to "hook" into tissue for lifting and tightening, and smooth threads, which add collagen and enhance skin texture without lifting. The techniques vary based on the material used (PDO, PLLA, or PCL), each with unique resorption timelines and effects on the skin.

To carry out a thread lift, the practitioner identifies key areas to insert and anchor the threads, based on the individual's facial structure and goals. Threads are typically inserted via a fine needle or cannula, which minimizes trauma to the tissue and provides precision. Once inserted, the threads are gently manipulated to ensure proper placement and achieve the desired lift and contour in the treated areas.

Over time, the body absorbs the threads, stimulating collagen production to maintain the lift and improved texture. Because different techniques can produce different results, practitioners may use varying approaches based on the client's skin laxity, target area, and preference. Thread lifts can effectively improve jawlines, and cheek contours, and even lift brows, providing a versatile approach to non-surgical facial rejuvenation.

Step-By-Step Guide To Thread Insertion Techniques

Thread insertion begins with careful facial mapping to mark the areas that require lifting. The skin is then cleansed and numbed with a topical anesthetic, allowing the procedure to be nearly painless. The practitioner uses fine needles or cannulas to insert threads at precise depths within the skin, following the pre-marked guides to ensure symmetry and the best aesthetic result.

Once the threads are in place, they are carefully pulled to achieve the desired lift. The practitioner smooths the skin over the threads, checking for an even, natural-looking result.

Lifting threads with barbs or hooks attach to soft tissue, lifting and holding it in position, while smooth threads are left intact without pulling, primarily to stimulate collagen.

After insertion, the area is gently massaged to secure the threads. Minor adjustments are made to avoid visible lumps or bumps, ensuring an even surface. The threads will integrate with the tissue as they are absorbed, and collagen production will gradually enhance firmness and smoothness, achieving a lifted appearance that lasts several months.

Differences Between Lifting And Smooth Threads

Lifting threads are designed with barbs, hooks, or cones that latch onto soft tissue, allowing the practitioner to reposition and lift sagging skin for an immediate tightening effect. These threads are often placed deeper within the skin to sustain the lifted appearance as long as possible. Lifting threads are commonly used for areas with more noticeable sagging, like the jawline and cheeks, where a defined contour is desired.

Smooth threads, on the other hand, are thin, straight, and lack the barbs needed for lifting. They are primarily used to improve skin texture and promote collagen production rather than to lift tissue. Smooth threads are typically placed in a mesh pattern, covering broader areas to stimulate collagen for a firming and rejuvenating effect. These threads are ideal for people looking for subtle, natural enhancements to skin texture rather than lifting.

In combining both thread types, practitioners can achieve dual effects—lifting and textural improvement—allowing for comprehensive facial rejuvenation. Selecting lifting or smooth threads depends on the patient's skin quality, desired outcome, and specific areas of focus, ensuring personalized and effective results.

Choosing The Right Technique For Different Facial Areas

Selecting the right thread lift technique for various facial areas depends on the skin's laxity and the desired lift. For instance, in the jawline, lifting threads are ideal for providing structure and definition, as the barbed threads can anchor and elevate sagging tissue.

In contrast, the delicate skin around the eyes and forehead may benefit more from smooth threads to stimulate collagen and improve texture without requiring heavy lifting.

For cheeks and mid-face areas, barbed lifting threads are often chosen to add volume and contour the cheekbones, providing a "lifted" appearance. Practitioners typically use a combination of lifting threads for primary support in the lower face and neck, while smooth threads can address fine lines and create smoother skin in thinner areas like the upper face and around the eyes.

The versatility of thread types allows practitioners to tailor the treatment to specific facial contours, balancing lift and rejuvenation based on individual needs.

This customization ensures each facial region receives appropriate treatment without overstretching or causing discomfort, maximizing results and satisfaction.

Combining Thread Lifts With Other Treatments (E.G., Fillers)

Combining thread lifts with dermal fillers can deliver enhanced and longer-lasting facial rejuvenation. Thread lifts provide structural support and lift, while fillers add volume to areas where fat loss or hollowing has occurred.

For example, in cases of volume loss in the cheeks, fillers can restore plumpness while the threads lift the skin, achieving a fuller and more youthful contour.

Botox is another complementary treatment that can be used alongside thread lifts. For instance, in the forehead and brow area, Botox can relax muscles that cause fine lines, while threads can help elevate sagging skin. Using these treatments together enhances the lift and smooths out the appearance of wrinkles for a more cohesive result.

Combining these treatments requires expertise to avoid "overfilling" or "over-lifting" the face. A well-planned combination strategy helps achieve a natural look by supporting the underlying structure with threads and adding volume or softening lines where needed, providing a more complete facial rejuvenation with minimal downtime.

Safety Tips To Avoid Common Complications During Insertion

Thread lifts are generally safe, but practitioners must take precautions to prevent complications like bruising, infection, or asymmetry.

First, using sterile instruments and disinfecting the skin properly before insertion is essential to reduce the risk of infection. A numbing cream or anesthetic is applied to minimize discomfort, allowing for smooth thread placement with less risk of tissue damage.

Selecting the appropriate thread type and insertion depth for each facial area helps prevent unwanted bumps, irregularities, or visible threads under the skin.

Practitioners are trained to monitor tension carefully to ensure an even lift and avoid over-pulling, which can lead to skin dimpling or puckering. Gentle handling of the threads during insertion and adjusting the tension as needed can prevent most aesthetic complications.

After the procedure, patients are advised to follow aftercare instructions, which often include avoiding strenuous activities and touching the treated areas for a few days. By taking these precautions, practitioners can help ensure a smooth recovery and effective, long-lasting results for thread lift patients.

CHAPTER FOUR

Anatomy Essentials For Thread Lifts

Thread lifts involve strategically placing dissolvable threads beneath the skin to provide lift and rejuvenation. To do this safely, a practitioner must have a strong understanding of facial anatomy, including key muscles, nerves, and blood vessels. Key muscles like the zygomaticus (cheek muscle) and orbicularis oculi (around the eyes) can affect how threads hold and distribute tension. Additionally, nerves such as the facial nerve and major vessels like the facial artery must be avoided to prevent pain, numbness, and bruising.

Threading must be performed in safe zones that allow for effective lifting without compromising essential facial structures. Safe areas generally include the jawline and the midface, where threads can work effectively with minimal risk.

However, certain regions—like around the temples, under-eye area, and near major nerve paths—pose higher risks for complications. The practitioner should mark these zones in advance and avoid threading too close to sensitive areas, maintaining a balance between effective lifting and safety.

Understanding skin tension and thread placement is essential for achieving optimal lift. The skin has natural tension lines, known as Langer's lines, that guide where threads should ideally be placed to provide the most natural results.

A skilled practitioner assesses the client's skin elasticity, facial shape, and bone structure to plan thread entry and exit points for the best outcome. This involves pre-visualizing the direction and anchoring points of each thread to ensure the lift is even and lasting.

Key Facial Muscles, Nerves, And Vessels To Consider

Key muscles involved in facial expressions, like the platysma (neck) and the levator labii (upper lip), play a role in how well thread lifts can reshape the face. The right placement near muscles like these can accentuate natural movements, giving a refreshed look without stiffness. Understanding how these muscles interact with skin tension also helps in making the lift appear natural and balanced.

Nerves, particularly the facial nerve, need careful navigation. The facial nerve divides into five branches across the face, controlling muscle movement. Any incorrect threading in these areas can result in numbness or, in rare cases, partial facial paralysis. Major arteries, like the facial artery and its branches, are equally critical to avoid, as threading near these could lead to significant bruising or hematoma.

Practitioners should pre-plan the threading path with these anatomical elements in mind, mapping out areas to avoid and others to focus on for lift and volume. This is typically done using markers to draw the expected placement on the face, creating a visual guide to work around key facial structures while ensuring a secure lift. Accurate placement around muscles and safe zones supports a better, safer outcome.

Safe Areas For Threading And Risk Zones To Avoid

Threading in safe areas is crucial to avoid complications. The jawline and mid-cheek areas are typically safer zones due to the lower risk of damaging critical vessels or nerves. These areas allow threads to grip firmly and lift the skin without hindering facial movement or risking serious side effects, providing effective results with fewer post-procedure issues.

Riskier zones include areas near the temples, around the eyes, and along the central forehead. These areas are more nerve-dense and near sensitive vascular paths, requiring skilled hands to avoid adverse effects. For example, the infraorbital area under the eyes is prone to swelling if mishandled, while the temple area has vital vessels that can bruise easily.

When performing thread lifts, practitioners often outline safe and risky areas beforehand to ensure proper placement. This pre-mapping technique provides a clear visual guide, helping to prevent accidental threading in risky regions.

By limiting threads to areas with fewer sensitive structures, practitioners minimize patient discomfort and enhance overall procedure safety.

Understanding Skin Tension And Thread Placement

Skin tension plays a fundamental role in the success of a thread lift. Langer's lines, the natural tension lines of the skin, serve as a roadmap for optimal thread placement, with threads ideally positioned along these lines to maximize lifting power. Following these lines ensures that the tension applied by the threads provides a natural look while supporting the skin's structure.

Thread placement involves planning entry and exit points on the face to create a balanced lift. Practitioners generally work from points that anchor the skin effectively, using specialized threads that either dissolve over time or stay in place depending on the result desired. This approach distributes lift evenly, avoiding an unnatural or over-pulled appearance. Each thread must be aligned with the skin's natural movement to integrate well with expressions.

By tailoring thread placement to each individual's skin tension and facial structure, practitioners can achieve harmonious results. Before insertion, they may test skin laxity by gently pinching the area to see how well it holds a lift. These adjustments ensure that each lift looks as seamless as possible, giving clients a refreshed appearance with minimal evidence of intervention.

How To Assess Client's Facial Structure For Optimal Results

A thorough facial assessment is crucial for effective thread lift outcomes. Practitioners start by analyzing the client's skin type, elasticity, and level of sagging in areas like the cheeks, jawline, and brows. This step identifies which areas will benefit most from a lift, allowing the practitioner to plan thread placements that complement the individual's natural contours.

Understanding the bone structure is also essential. Bone support varies across individuals, affecting how threads will anchor and hold.

For example, people with high cheekbones may require fewer threads in the midface, while those with a flatter profile might need more structural support. This evaluation often includes a discussion of the client's aesthetic goals to ensure the treatment aligns with their expectations and facial anatomy.

Lastly, symmetry and balance are evaluated, as thread lifts aim to enhance these features subtly. The practitioner may use measurements or visual markers to align threads with specific points on the face, ensuring an even lift across both sides. This personalized assessment helps the practitioner tailor the thread lift to create natural, symmetrical, and long-lasting results.

Importance Of Post-Procedure Anatomical Review

After completing the procedure, practitioners conduct a post-procedure anatomical review to ensure the threads are secure and correctly positioned. This step involves gentle palpation and visual assessment to confirm that no threads are visible on the skin surface and that the lift is even. Anomalies like bunching or visible threads are immediately corrected to avoid later complications.

Assessing any signs of swelling or bruising is crucial, as these are natural responses but should be monitored to avoid excessive discomfort. The practitioner may advise gentle massaging techniques, where appropriate, to reduce minor swelling or to help the threads settle into place more smoothly. This helps the client achieve a smoother, more comfortable healing process.

Clear aftercare instructions, such as avoiding strenuous activity and refraining from pulling on the skin, support a successful recovery. The practitioner will typically review the results after a few days to check thread positioning and address any client concerns. This ongoing anatomical assessment and support ensure that clients get the best possible results from their thread lift therapy.

CHAPTER FIVE

Post-Procedure Care And Client Instructions

After a thread lift, it's essential to follow specific care instructions to support recovery and achieve optimal results. Immediately after the procedure, keep the treated area clean and avoid touching it unnecessarily to prevent any irritation.

Use mild, lukewarm water to gently cleanse the skin, and refrain from applying makeup for at least 24 hours. Elevating your head while sleeping can help reduce swelling, and using a cold compress in the first 24-48 hours can also alleviate discomfort and minimize puffiness.

Immediate Post-Procedure Care Tips

In the initial days post-procedure, avoid any intense facial movements and be mindful when speaking, laughing, or chewing. To prevent infection, avoid touching or pressing on the treated area, and do not sleep on your stomach or side to avoid pressure on the threads. It's recommended to avoid alcohol, caffeine, and smoking for the first few days, as these can contribute to inflammation and slow down the healing process. Use only prescribed or recommended topical ointments, avoiding products with strong active ingredients.

Handling Common Side Effects: Swelling, Bruising, Etc

Swelling, bruising, and some soreness are normal and should subside within a few days to a week. If swelling persists, applying ice packs intermittently in short 10-minute sessions can provide relief. Bruising may take a week or more to fade and can be covered with light makeup after the initial 24 hours. To relieve any discomfort, over-the-counter pain medications can be used unless contraindicated by your provider. If you experience any severe pain, oozing, or unusual symptoms, reach out to your practitioner immediately.

Long-Term Care Guidelines For Sustained Results

Long-term care is crucial to maintain the effects of the thread lift. Regular moisturizing and sun protection help keep the skin in good condition and prolong the lift's impact. SPF 30 or higher is essential for protecting the skin, as UV rays can accelerate skin aging.

Incorporate gentle, hydrating products, and avoid skincare with harsh chemicals or exfoliants for at least a month. Some clients may also consider mild, supportive treatments, such as collagen-boosting facials, as advised by their practitioner, to enhance the results.

Activity Restrictions And Skin Care Tips Post-Thread Lift

For the first week post-procedure, avoid strenuous activities, including exercise, as it may displace the threads or increase bruising. Refrain from any activity that increases blood flow to the face, such as saunas, hot tubs, or steam rooms. Avoid massaging or applying direct pressure to the face during this period, and switch to gentle skincare, steering clear of scrubs, peels, and acids until your provider gives the all-clear. Stick to a mild cleanser and a fragrance-free moisturizer, allowing the skin to recover fully.

Follow-Up Consultation And Ongoing Assessment Schedule

Follow-up appointments are generally scheduled about one week after the procedure to monitor healing and assess for any side effects. During these visits, your provider can address any concerns and recommend additional care, if necessary. Subsequent follow-ups may occur at one month and three months to ensure the threads are settling well and delivering the desired lift.

Maintenance appointments, if needed, can be discussed during these consultations based on individual progress and goals.

CHAPTER SIX

Managing Common Concerns And Complications

Thread lifts are minimally invasive, but certain concerns can arise, such as swelling, bruising, or mild discomfort post-procedure. Proper aftercare, including applying cold compresses, avoiding intense physical activity, and keeping the treated area elevated, can significantly reduce these issues. Patients are advised not to rub or manipulate the area excessively to avoid disturbing the threads.

Complications such as thread migration or visible lumps might occasionally occur. A skilled practitioner can address these by adjusting the threads manually, using specialized tools, or, in rare cases, removing or repositioning the thread entirely. Monitoring recovery closely during the first few days is essential to ensure the threads settle properly.

To minimize risks, it's crucial to follow aftercare instructions diligently. Regular check-ins with the doctor can help detect early complications and resolve them quickly. Patients should avoid blood-thinning medications and alcohol before and after treatment to reduce the chances of excessive bruising or swelling.

Identifying And Addressing Asymmetry Issues

Asymmetry can occur if the threads are not placed symmetrically or if one side of the face heals differently. Practitioners need to mark the insertion points carefully and assess the patient's facial structure before starting the procedure. Minor asymmetries may also become more noticeable after swelling subsides, so waiting a few weeks to evaluate the final result is important.

If the asymmetry is detected, adjustments can be made by either tightening or loosening specific threads to create a more balanced appearance. In some cases, additional threads may need to be inserted to provide the desired correction. These touch-up treatments are often quick and require minimal downtime.

Patients should communicate any concerns about unevenness during follow-up appointments. Practitioners may suggest additional contouring procedures, such as dermal fillers, to complement the thread lift results and achieve facial symmetry if needed.

Infection Prevention And Treatment Steps

Infections are rare but possible if proper hygiene isn't maintained. To prevent this, practitioners must use sterile tools, and patients should thoroughly clean the skin before the procedure. Antibiotic creams or oral antibiotics may be prescribed as a preventive measure.

After the procedure, patients should avoid touching the treated area unnecessarily and follow instructions on keeping the insertion points clean and dry. If any redness, warmth, or pus appears, it might indicate an infection, which should be addressed immediately by the medical team.

In case of an infection, early treatment with prescribed antibiotics usually resolves the issue without complications. In severe cases, the affected thread may need to be removed to prevent further spread. Regular follow-ups help detect any signs of infection early and ensure timely intervention.

Managing Discomfort And Pain Relief Options

Thread lifts usually cause mild discomfort rather than severe pain, with most patients feeling tightness or a slight pulling sensation for a few days. Over-the-counter pain relievers like acetaminophen or ibuprofen are commonly recommended to alleviate any post-procedural soreness.

Cold compresses can reduce both pain and swelling during the first 24 hours after treatment. Patients are encouraged to avoid vigorous facial movements, such as laughing or chewing hard foods, during the initial recovery phase to minimize discomfort.

If pain persists beyond a few days or worsens, it's important to contact the provider. They may prescribe stronger pain medications or adjust the threads if they are irritating. Proper aftercare and rest are crucial in ensuring smooth recovery and minimizing discomfort.

Addressing Thread Visibility Or Migration Concerns

Thread visibility, such as seeing or feeling the threads under the skin, can sometimes occur, especially if the skin is thin or the placement is too shallow. Skilled practitioners aim to place threads deep enough to avoid this issue, but slight irregularities might still arise.

If threads become visible or migrate, minor adjustments can usually correct the issue. The practitioner can gently massage the area to reposition the thread or cut the protruding end if necessary. In some cases, dissolvable threads may naturally break down and become less noticeable over time.

To avoid migration, patients should refrain from intense facial movements, sleeping on the face, or applying pressure to the treated area. It's also important to attend follow-up sessions so the practitioner can monitor thread placement and make timely corrections.

Steps To Handle Emergency Situations Safely

Emergencies, though rare, may include excessive bleeding, allergic reactions, or sudden swelling. Patients should know what signs to watch for, such as difficulty breathing or severe pain, and contact their provider immediately if these occur.

If excessive bleeding happens at the insertion points, applying pressure with a clean cloth can help slow it down while waiting for medical attention. In case of an allergic reaction, such as hives or difficulty breathing, antihistamines or epinephrine might be required. Always have emergency contacts and medications available.

To handle emergencies safely, both practitioners and patients must have a post-procedure action plan. This includes having emergency supplies ready and ensuring patients understand when to seek immediate care. Regular communication with the medical team can help resolve most issues promptly.

CHAPTER SEVEN

Advanced Techniques For Optimal Results

In thread lift therapy, advanced techniques are designed to enhance and refine results beyond standard procedures. One effective approach is using various insertion angles and thread placements to target specific facial contours, such as lifting the jawline or enhancing cheekbones.

Angling threads in different directions can provide a balanced lift, helping avoid an overly taut or unnatural look. These techniques allow practitioners to contour specific areas more precisely, optimizing results for the patient's unique facial structure.

To maximize results, practitioners can combine different types of threads, such as mono threads for volume and barbed threads for lift. Mono threads add subtle plumpness to sunken areas, while barbed threads secure a lift, particularly around the brows, cheeks, and jawline. The combination of thread types in a single treatment session can improve overall facial symmetry, making the approach highly customizable based on individual aesthetic needs.

Layering threads at different depths is also beneficial, especially for patients with thicker skin or more pronounced sagging. In these cases, layering supports the structure of the face and can provide long-lasting results. It's crucial that this layering be done skillfully to avoid overloading the skin. Practitioners should consider the thickness and texture of the skin to prevent complications and ensure a smooth, youthful appearance.

Combination Treatments To Enhance Thread Lift Results

Combining thread lifts with other aesthetic treatments, such as dermal fillers or botulinum toxin, can significantly enhance results. Fillers are often used alongside thread lifts to provide additional volume to areas such as the cheeks or lips, enhancing the lift effect and creating a fuller appearance. This combination allows for immediate volume boost and long-term lifting, addressing both sagging and volume loss simultaneously.

Laser and radiofrequency (RF) treatments are also excellent complements to thread lifts, as they help to tighten the skin and boost collagen production post-procedure.

When used after a thread lift, RF treatments can firm the skin, helping threads work more effectively and prolong the tightening effects. Laser treatments can help improve skin texture and tone, which, when combined with a lift, gives a completely rejuvenated look.

Chemical peels or microneedling can be used in combination with thread lifts to refine skin texture. These treatments help minimize fine lines, reduce pigmentation, and provide a fresh, radiant glow. The combination of a thread lift with resurfacing treatments allows for both structural and surface-level improvements, enhancing the overall outcome and ensuring a more comprehensive rejuvenation.

Using Different Thread Types Together For Custom Results

Practitioners often use various thread types together in a single session to achieve specific aesthetic goals. For example, PDO (polydioxanone) threads, commonly used for their collagen-stimulating properties, can be paired with PLLA (poly-L-lactic acid) threads, which provide longer-lasting lifting effects. This combination allows practitioners to use PDO threads for subtle collagen stimulation while PLLA threads provide sustained lift, ideal for areas needing prolonged support.

Cogs or barbed threads are frequently combined with smooth or mono threads in a single session. Barbed threads have hooks or barbs that anchor the skin for lifting, while mono threads provide slight volumizing, filling in areas that may appear sunken. This combined approach can lift while restoring lost volume, producing a more balanced and natural look, particularly effective for mid-face rejuvenation and jawline definition.

Different thread materials such as PCL (polycaprolactone) can also be mixed with PDO and PLLA for customized effects. PCL threads dissolve more slowly, making them suitable for patients desiring a longer-lasting lift. Customizing thread materials based on the patient's needs helps ensure an individualized treatment plan and results tailored to specific facial anatomy and aging concerns.

Layering And Angling Techniques For Specific Effects

Layering and angling techniques in thread lift therapy provide additional control over the lift and contour effects. When layering, threads are inserted at various depths and locations, which can improve both support and durability. For instance, placing deeper threads offers foundational support, while superficial threads provide surface lift, ideal for enhancing high-precision areas such as around the eyes and mouth.

Angling techniques allow practitioners to direct the lift in particular directions, targeting specific areas like the brow, cheekbones, or jawline. Angling threads upward toward the temples can lift sagging brows, while horizontal threads along the jawline help in defining facial contours. Skilled angling is especially useful for patients with asymmetrical facial features, enabling practitioners to balance these areas with precision.

Layering with various thread types further enhances the customization of effects. Using a combination of barbed and mono threads in different layers offers a multi-dimensional lift, supporting areas of sagging while adding volume.

Practitioners often utilize specific anchoring points on the face to ensure that the layered threads work together harmoniously, creating results that feel both natural and structured.

Expert Tips On Tightening And Volumizing Approaches

Experienced practitioners often focus on a dual approach of tightening and volumizing to achieve a balanced rejuvenation. Tightening is generally accomplished using barbed or cog threads to lift the skin, providing immediate support to sagging areas. For volumizing, mono or smooth threads are used to fill in hollow regions like the cheeks or temples. This combined technique offers both structural lift and softness, essential for a natural look.

When tightening around the jawline, the direction of the lift plays a significant role in achieving a defined contour.

Practitioners typically anchor threads near the ears or temples to pull the jawline upward and outward, enhancing facial shape without appearing overdone. Proper insertion angles ensure a firm, lifted effect, particularly effective in enhancing the youthful "V-shape" face.

For volumizing, mono threads can be inserted in a grid pattern over areas like the cheeks or nasolabial folds to create subtle fullness and smooth lines.

Expert practitioners carefully monitor the amount of thread used, as over-volumizing can lead to puffiness rather than a natural look.

The combination of targeted tightening and gentle volumizing brings a balanced effect that both lifts and refreshes the face, tailored to the patient's aesthetic goals.

Case Studies On Advanced Thread Lift Applications

Case studies show the versatility and adaptability of advanced thread lift applications in meeting diverse patient needs. For example, a 50-year-old woman seeking mid-face rejuvenation with subtle cheek contouring might benefit from a combination of barbed and mono threads.

In this case, the practitioner used barbed threads to lift the mid-face and mono threads for subtle volume, resulting in a natural lift without excessive fullness.

Another case involved a male patient in his late 40s with moderate jawline sagging and minimal cheek volume loss.

The practitioner used long, barbed threads anchored near the temples to lift the jawline, combined with a few mono threads along the cheeks. This approach subtly lifted the jawline and maintained a masculine contour while adding minimal volume, showcasing how thread lifts can be customized based on gender-specific aesthetics.

For patients with more significant sagging, layering techniques were employed. A woman in her 60s, for instance, received barbed threads at a deeper layer for lift and mono threads at a superficial layer for fine-tuning volume.

This layering approach improved both structural support and skin surface texture, leading to a comprehensive rejuvenation. These case studies illustrate the adaptability of thread lifts to different facial structures, aging patterns, and personal preferences.

CHAPTER EIGHT

Client Care Strategies And Communication

Building Client Trust Through Clear Communication

To foster trust with clients undergoing thread lift therapy, practitioners must focus on transparent, approachable communication. Clients should feel comfortable discussing their concerns, questions, and expectations from the very first consultation.

Using open-ended questions allows clients to express their aesthetic goals fully and provides practitioners with the insight needed to tailor the treatment plan accordingly. Developing rapport through active listening and empathy will set a foundation for trust, enabling clients to feel confident in the practitioner's expertise.

Consistently updating clients about each stage of the thread lift procedure can demystify the process and ease any anxieties. Educate clients on what they can expect before, during, and after the procedure. Take time to discuss the healing process, anticipated results, and the timeline for visible improvements, ensuring clients have a realistic understanding of what will occur. When practitioners communicate with care and precision, clients are more likely to feel secure and satisfied with their decisions.

Following the procedure, scheduling follow-up appointments, or sending out check-in messages shows a commitment to client well-being and recovery. Offer clients accessible channels to reach out if they have questions post-treatment. Making time for these follow-ups not only ensures the client feels valued but also allows practitioners to address any potential complications promptly. This approach to aftercare supports client satisfaction and enhances the overall experience, increasing the likelihood of future referrals and a positive reputation.

Explaining Benefits And Limitations Effectively

Thread lifts offer unique benefits, such as lifting and tightening the skin without the need for invasive surgery. To ensure clients understand these advantages, practitioners should present them in an easily comprehensible manner.

Explain that the procedure involves the use of dissolvable sutures that are inserted under the skin to create a lifted appearance, and discuss how these threads stimulate collagen production over time, promoting a more youthful look. Emphasizing the quick recovery period and minimal downtime can reassure clients seeking subtle rejuvenation.

Equally important is outlining the limitations of thread lift therapy. Make it clear that while thread lifts can achieve significant skin-tightening effects, they are not suitable for everyone, particularly those with very advanced skin laxity or significant volume loss. In these cases, a surgical facelift may be a more effective option. By being upfront about the constraints, practitioners help manage client expectations and avoid potential disappointment with the results.

Clients should also be aware of potential side effects or complications, such as minor bruising, swelling, or thread visibility, which can occur temporarily. Discussing these potential risks openly can prepare clients and build their confidence in the practitioner's honesty and competence. A well-informed client is more likely to have a satisfying experience and a better understanding of the outcome.

Answering Common Client Questions About Results And Risks

Clients often come with numerous questions about how thread lift results will look and any associated risks.

A common question is about the duration of the results, which usually last 12 to 18 months.

Practitioners should explain that the threads gradually dissolve over time, leaving behind collagen that continues to support the skin, which is why maintenance treatments are recommended every year or so for prolonged results. By clearly explaining this process, clients can better appreciate the longevity of their treatment.

Clients may also ask about immediate results versus longer-term effects. It is essential to explain that while some lifting is visible right after the procedure, full results appear gradually as the collagen builds.

Additionally, addressing any misconceptions about risks—such as fears of facial asymmetry or "over-pulled" appearances—can reassure clients. Emphasize that thread lifts, when done by skilled practitioners, yield natural, subtle improvements.

Finally, clients may inquire about potential complications and how these are managed. Practitioners should go over possible side effects like mild bruising, swelling, and rare cases of infection, emphasizing that these are manageable with appropriate post-care. Providing reassurance about the safety and reversibility of thread lifts (as the threads dissolve naturally) can further alleviate client anxiety, making the decision process smoother.

Managing Expectations For Realistic Outcomes

A key aspect of client satisfaction in thread lift therapy is helping clients set realistic expectations for their results. Practitioners should emphasize that thread lifts provide subtle, natural-looking enhancements rather than drastic transformations. Show clients examples of before-and-after photos from previous procedures to give them a tangible sense of the kind of improvements they can expect. This helps align the client's expectations with achievable results, preventing misunderstandings post-procedure.

Discussing the gradual improvement process is crucial, as clients may expect instant transformation.

Practitioners should clarify that while initial lifting can be seen immediately, collagen stimulation and skin tightening develop gradually over a few months. Being transparent about this timeline can keep clients patient and reduce disappointment if immediate changes aren't as dramatic as expected.

Setting expectations for maintenance is also essential. Thread lifts are semi-permanent and typically require touch-ups every 12 to 18 months to maintain the effects. By explaining that results naturally diminish as threads dissolve, clients are better prepared for the long-term commitment of the treatment. When expectations are managed thoughtfully, clients are more likely to appreciate the results and remain satisfied with their decisions.

Ensuring Client Satisfaction And Follow-Up Support

Providing exceptional follow-up support is essential for ensuring client satisfaction with their thread lift therapy. Aftercare plays a significant role in the client's overall experience and can significantly impact how they perceive the procedure's effectiveness.

Practitioners should schedule a post-treatment consultation to assess the client's recovery, answer questions, and confirm that they are satisfied with their results. These interactions reinforce the practitioner's commitment to the client's well-being.

CHAPTER NINE

Common FAQs For Thread Lift Practitioners

What Types Of Results Can Clients Expect?

Clients can expect a noticeable but subtle lift in the areas treated, which can include the cheeks, jawline, neck, or brows. Unlike more invasive surgical lifts, thread lifts offer a more natural effect that enhances facial contours without a "pulled" appearance.

Results also depend on the specific type of thread used, the areas targeted, and the client's skin condition. Most patients report a firmer, tighter appearance immediately following the procedure, with further improvements as collagen production increases in the months after.

Over the next few weeks, the body begins to produce more collagen around the threads, which enhances skin elasticity and gives the face a more youthful, rejuvenated look. The lifting effect gradually becomes more prominent as the skin tightens naturally. Thread lifts are typically best suited for mild to moderate sagging and can significantly improve the overall facial structure of clients who are not ready for a surgical facelift.

Some clients may notice initial swelling or slight bruising, which generally fades within a week. As the threads settle into place, the results become more subtle, and most clients achieve an optimal look within one to three months. This natural improvement makes thread lifts popular among clients looking for low-downtime, gradual results without drastic changes in appearance.

How Long Do Thread Lift Results Typically Last?

The longevity of thread lift results varies, but generally, clients can expect results to last between one to three years, depending on the type of thread used and individual factors like skin quality, age, and lifestyle.

PDO (Polydioxanone) threads, for instance, typically dissolve within 6-12 months, while PLLA (Poly-L-Lactic Acid) and PCL (Polycaprolactone) threads may last longer, up to 18-24 months. Even after the threads dissolve, the collagen generated in response to the threads can help maintain some lifting effects.

Clients looking for longer-lasting results can consider combining thread lifts with other treatments, such as fillers or PRP therapy, which can complement the lifting effect by adding volume and improving skin quality. Regular skincare, sun protection, and avoiding lifestyle factors like smoking can also extend the longevity of the results.

For optimal, longer-lasting effects, some clients may opt for periodic thread lift maintenance treatments every 12-18 months. Practitioners typically reassess results during follow-up visits and make personalized recommendations based on the client's aging patterns and aesthetic goals.

Are There Risks Of Allergic Reactions To Threads?

Thread lift materials are generally biocompatible, meaning they are designed to be well-tolerated by the body and unlikely to cause allergic reactions. PDO, PLLA, and PCL threads are all FDA-approved for use in aesthetic treatments and are known for their safety profiles. However, as with any foreign material, there is a small risk of sensitivity or allergy, particularly if a client has a history of reactions to similar materials.

To minimize risk, practitioners should conduct a thorough consultation, including a client's medical history and any previous adverse reactions to materials like sutures. In rare cases, clients may experience a mild inflammatory response, which is usually manageable with over-the-counter anti-inflammatory medication and subsides quickly.

If a client experiences persistent discomfort, redness, or swelling after the procedure, it may indicate an allergic response or other complication, and they should consult with their practitioner promptly. However, adverse reactions are generally minimal and manageable with proper technique and post-care.

Can Thread Lifts Be Done Alongside Other Facial Treatments?

Yes, thread lifts can be safely combined with other facial treatments for more comprehensive facial rejuvenation. Many clients choose to complement thread lifts with dermal fillers to add volume or with botulinum toxin (Botox) to smooth dynamic wrinkles. This combination is often referred to as a "liquid facelift," offering the dual benefits of lifting and volumizing without surgery.

For safety, practitioners should space out certain treatments. For instance, dermal fillers are often administered a few weeks after the thread lift to allow the threads to settle. Non-invasive skin treatments like chemical peels, microneedling, and radiofrequency are generally safe when done before or after a thread lift, although timing should be carefully managed to minimize skin sensitivity and maximize results.

Clients should discuss their goals with their practitioner, who will provide a customized treatment plan that balances the timing of multiple procedures. Combined treatments can yield enhanced results, often allowing clients to achieve a more youthful, refreshed appearance in fewer sessions.

What Are The Signs Of Potential Complications?

Thread lifts are generally safe with minimal downtime, but, like any procedure, they come with potential risks. Common side effects include temporary swelling, bruising, and mild discomfort, which usually resolve on their own within a few days to a week.

However, clients and practitioners should be aware of signs of complications that may require further intervention. Signs of complications include severe pain, redness that worsens over time, noticeable asymmetry, and visible threads poking through the skin. Infection, though rare, is another possible complication and may present as redness, warmth, or discharge at the thread insertion points. Clients experiencing these symptoms should contact their practitioner promptly for evaluation.

In cases where threads migrate or the skin pulls unevenly, corrective treatments may be necessary. Thread visibility is uncommon when the procedure is performed correctly, but in rare instances, threads may need to be adjusted or removed if they become noticeable. Proper post-care, like avoiding vigorous facial movements and heavy exercise, can help minimize complications.

CHAPTER TEN

Industry Insights And Best Practices

Thread lifts have become a popular non-surgical facelift solution, offering a minimally invasive alternative to traditional surgery. The process involves using absorbable threads that are inserted under the skin to lift sagging tissues, providing a subtle and natural rejuvenation. Best practices in this industry focus on using high-quality materials like PDO (Polydioxanone) threads and ensuring patient safety through proper hygiene and procedural care. Practitioners must follow strict protocols for thread placement and aftercare to prevent complications and enhance results.

Ensuring that thread lifts are performed by skilled and certified professionals is another key aspect of best practices. Proper knowledge of facial anatomy, thread insertion techniques, and an understanding of skin types are vital for achieving optimal outcomes. Clinics that prioritize ongoing staff training and maintaining up-to-date licenses are more likely to achieve successful patient results and build trust within the community.

Lastly, patient consultation plays a critical role in best practices. Thorough discussions about client expectations, realistic outcomes, and possible side effects should be addressed before the procedure. Providing detailed aftercare instructions and follow-up appointments helps ensure a smooth recovery and long-lasting results, keeping patient satisfaction high.

Current Trends In Non-Surgical Facelifting

The aesthetic industry is seeing a surge in demand for non-surgical facelifting solutions, with thread lifts being at the forefront of this trend. Patients are drawn to thread lifts because of the minimal downtime, less invasive nature, and the ability to achieve natural-looking results. Current trends include the use of advanced PDO threads that not only lift but also stimulate collagen production, further enhancing the skin's texture and elasticity over time.

One notable trend is the customization of thread lift treatments. Clinics are now tailoring procedures to meet individual needs, whether it's a full facelift, mid-face lift, or localized treatments for areas like the neck or jawline.

This personalized approach ensures that clients get the most out of their thread lifts without the risks associated with more invasive surgeries.

Another trend gaining popularity is the combination of thread lifts with other non-invasive procedures, such as dermal fillers or skin resurfacing treatments. By layering these techniques, practitioners can offer comprehensive anti-aging solutions that deliver more dramatic and long-lasting results, catering to the growing demand for subtle, yet effective cosmetic enhancements.

Certification And Training For Thread Lift Practitioners

Becoming a certified thread lift practitioner requires specialized training to ensure practitioners are well-equipped with the skills needed to perform the procedure safely and effectively. Training programs often include both theoretical and practical components, covering essential topics such as facial anatomy, thread insertion techniques, and managing potential complications. Aspiring practitioners must undergo hands-on experience under the supervision of experienced mentors before they can be certified.

Certification programs typically involve learning how to select the right type of thread for different skin types and areas of the face. Practitioners must also be trained in proper sterilization methods, anesthesia administration, and patient consultation techniques to ensure the highest level of care. Many certification programs offer ongoing education to help practitioners stay updated on the latest advancements and techniques in the industry.

Upon completion of training, practitioners are awarded a certification that is recognized by professional bodies in the aesthetic field. This certification not only validates their expertise but also instills confidence in potential clients who are seeking safe, professional care.

Regular recertification and additional training are recommended as new technologies and products emerge in the field of non-surgical facelifts.

Ethical Practices In Aesthetic Procedures

Ethical practices in aesthetic procedures, including thread lifts, are essential to ensuring patient safety and maintaining trust in the industry.

Practitioners must prioritize patient well-being over profit by providing honest assessments of what the procedure can achieve and setting realistic expectations. This includes turning away clients who may not be good candidates for thread lifts due to medical reasons or unrealistic expectations about the results.

Informed consent is a fundamental aspect of ethical practice. Practitioners must provide comprehensive information about the risks, benefits, potential side effects, and the recovery process associated with thread lifts.

This transparency allows patients to make educated decisions about their treatment, minimizing the risk of dissatisfaction or post-procedure complications.

Another ethical consideration is the importance of proper aftercare. Practitioners are responsible for providing patients with clear instructions on how to care for their skin after the procedure and should offer follow-up appointments to monitor recovery.

Ethical practices also extend to maintaining privacy and confidentiality, ensuring that patient information is protected and treated with respect.

Tips For Growing A Successful Aesthetic Practice

Building a successful aesthetic practice in the thread lift industry requires a combination of clinical expertise, excellent customer service, and smart marketing strategies. First, providing exceptional results is key—investing in high-quality products, staying up-to-date with the latest techniques, and continually improving skills will ensure client satisfaction and foster word-of-mouth referrals. Aesthetic practitioners who prioritize patient safety and deliver natural-looking outcomes are more likely to build a loyal customer base.

Another critical tip is to invest in staff training and customer service. Clients appreciate being treated with professionalism, care, and respect from the moment they step into the clinic.

Having a well-trained team that is knowledgeable about the procedures, able to answer client questions, and create a welcoming environment will enhance the overall experience and encourage repeat business.

Marketing your practice effectively is also essential for growth. Developing a strong online presence through social media, showcasing before-and-after results, and engaging with potential clients through educational content can help attract new business. Offering special promotions or referral programs can also incentivize clients to spread the word about your services, helping to expand your practice organically.

Continuous Learning And Staying Updated

The aesthetic industry, including thread lifts, is rapidly evolving, making continuous learning an essential part of any practitioner's career. Staying informed about new products, techniques, and technologies can help practitioners offer the best possible care to their clients. Attending conferences, workshops, and certification courses regularly ensures that practitioners are up to date with the latest trends and advancements in the field.

Networking with other professionals in the industry also provides valuable learning opportunities. By connecting with peers, practitioners can share insights, learn from each other's experiences, and discuss industry challenges. This collaborative approach to learning can open doors to new ideas and approaches that may enhance a practitioner's skills and improve patient outcomes.

Finally, investing in ongoing education is not just about technical skills—it also involves staying updated on the latest regulations, ethical considerations, and patient care standards.

By committing to continuous learning, practitioners not only improve their expertise but also help elevate the overall standard of care in the industry, leading to safer and more effective treatments for patients.

Conclusion

Thread lift therapy, as a non-surgical cosmetic procedure, has gained popularity for its ability to achieve subtle, natural-looking facial rejuvenation with minimal downtime. This treatment involves the insertion of dissolvable sutures under the skin to lift and tighten sagging tissues. Thread lifts offer a versatile solution for patients seeking an alternative to traditional facelift surgeries, as they are minimally invasive, allowing faster recovery and fewer side effects.

One of the most significant benefits of thread lifts is their dual-action approach: not only do they lift sagging skin, but they also stimulate collagen production, leading to a gradual improvement in skin texture and elasticity over time. The threads used in these procedures typically dissolve within six months; however, the effects can last up to two years due to the body's natural healing and collagen-boosting responses.

While thread lift therapy offers several advantages, it is essential to set realistic expectations. This procedure is ideal for mild to moderate sagging; individuals with more significant signs of aging may not achieve their desired results solely from a thread lift. Additionally, like all cosmetic procedures, thread lifts carry potential risks, such as infection, scarring, or asymmetry, although these are rare with a qualified professional.

In conclusion, thread lift therapy presents a compelling option for individuals seeking subtle rejuvenation without the need for surgery. By promoting collagen production and lifting sagging areas, thread lifts offer lasting benefits and natural-looking results. As technology and techniques advance, the effectiveness and safety of thread lifts continue to improve.

However, consulting with a qualified practitioner is essential for achieving optimal results and ensuring that thread lifts align with individual aesthetic goals. This treatment can be a valuable addition to a broader skincare or anti-aging routine, providing a low-risk option for enhancing one's natural appearance.

THE END

www.ingramcontent.com/pod-product-compliance
Lightning Source LLC
Chambersburg PA
CBHW061052250726
48653CB00001B/361

9 798300 775261